YOGA
of
Courage
and
Compassion

"This is a brave and passionate book that should be in every yoga lover's backpack. It shows that yoga is far more than the beneficial physical exercise it has often been reduced to in our materialist culture, and it demonstrates with precise verve how doing yoga can provide a foundation of galvanized yet peaceful energy for the courageous work of sacred activism and for rising gracefully to the brutal challenges of our time."

ANDREW HARVEY,
COAUTHOR OF *HEART YOGA*

"There is more to yoga than staying limber, youthful, and healthy. The confrontation with the vulnerability of the body and the finite nature of life is an essential moment of spiritual learning. William Yang has collected precious lessons about courage, compassion, and love in the years he has worked with people who have cancer. He has brought these lessons together in this book, opening up a deeper dimension in yoga. His exercises are simple, yet profound and very energetic. They help you embrace the totality of life and enjoy the depth of the moment. William's work has become a source of inspiration for many yoga teachers and their students. I can heartily recommend this book."

LEA VOS, FORMER DIRECTOR OF ZWEIERSDAL,
CENTER FOR YOGA AND CONTINUING EDUCATION
FOR YOGA TEACHERS

"William Yang invites people to take the journey into the depth of their own being. If people are willing to investigate their life in the face of death, all false solutions will be destroyed. This book is not only for the sick but for all those affected by the incurable disease of life. *Yoga of Courage and Compassion* is remarkable."

DRS. NOL HOGEMA, OP, FORMER DIRECTOR
OF THE HAN FORTMAN CENTER

YOGA
of Courage
and Compassion

Conscious Breathing and Guided Meditation

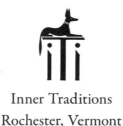

A Sacred Planet Book

William Yang

Inner Traditions

Rochester, Vermont

Inner Traditions
One Park Street
Rochester, Vermont 05767
www.InnerTraditions.com

Sacred Planet Books are curated by Richard Grossinger, Inner Traditions editorial board member and cofounder and former publisher of North Atlantic Books. The Sacred Planet collection, published under the umbrella of the Inner Traditions family of imprints, is comprised of works on the themes of consciousness, cosmology, alternative medicine, dreams, climate, permaculture, alchemy, shamanic studies, oracles, astrology, crystals, hyperobjects, locutions, and subtle bodies.

Originally published in Dutch under the title *Yoga van moed en mededogen* by
    Taborhuis, Nijmeegsebaan 27, 6561 KE Groesbeek, Netherlands
First U.S. edition published in 2021 by Inner Traditions

Note to the reader: This book is intended as an informational guide. The remedies, approaches, and techniques described herein are meant to supplement, and not to be a substitute for, professional medical care or treatment. They should not be used to treat a serious ailment without prior consultation with a qualified health care professional.

Cataloging-in-Publication Data for this title is available from the Library of Congress

ISBN 978-1-64411-286-1 (print)
ISBN 978-1-64411-287-8 (ebook)

Printed and bound in the United States by Versa Press, Inc.

10 9 8 7 6 5 4 3 2 1

Text design by Priscilla Baker and layout by VirginiaScott Bowman
This book was typeset in Garamond Premier Pro and Futura with Bell used as the display typface
Artwork by Karen van der Pas

To send correspondence to the author of this book, mail a first-class letter to the author c/o Inner Traditions • Bear & Company, One Park Street, Rochester, VT 05767, and we will forward the communication, or contact the author directly at **w.yang@williamyang.nl**.

Contents

Introduction

The German philosopher Friedrich Nietzsche once said that he wanted to write philosophy with a hammer. Likewise, I would like to teach yoga with a hammer. With a hammer and a sword, even! A hammer to break, and a sword to cut through the walls and fundaments of the ego-centered mind, but with tenderness and compassion, to touch the ego's vulnerability and challenge its defensiveness and its desperately cherished "peace of mind."

This special kind of yoga was developed through the years I worked with people who had cancer and their relatives. In 1983 I was invited to implement a counseling program for cancer patients in the Canisius Wilhelmina Hospital in Nijmegen, eastern Netherlands. Inspired by the pioneering work of oncologist Dr. O. Carl Simonton in the 1970s, this program integrated a variety of body-mind techniques to give patients effective tools to "fight for their lives" by stimulating the power of the mind over the body.

And it worked. Many patients were able to mobilize and enhance their healing process and not rely only on doctors and medicine. Of course, not every patient was physically

1

cured, but many appreciated gaining a clearly discernible influence over their quality of life by gaining a more realistic control over their thoughts, feelings, and communications. They reported feeling better, sleeping better, and having a more positive outlook on life.

But it seldom worked completely.

The power of an illness that uproots the foundations of life itself and all its dreams, plans, and expectations is greater than any body-mind technique. All the benefits of the exercises I so patiently taught could be hammered down and cut through overnight by the brutal force of cancer. This enemy shattered all defense barriers.

The proverb "If you can't beat 'em, join 'em" applies to cancer. So in the end many cancer patients were forced to do the unimaginable: join the overwhelming force of the cancer instead of resisting it, letting it become an ally. Rather than putting up a last frenetic fight against this enemy, patients began to give in to it and let go of the fighting. They realized that tenacious clinging to dear life would get them nowhere. They learned to relax somehow, to rest and allow the mind to become still. This stilling of the mind requires inordinate courage, especially as it requires accepting life as it is: impermanent.

Impermanence is the bedrock of the Buddha's teachings, and was the shocking truth that Jesus Christ demonstrated through his own vulnerable human life and death.

Peace of mind in the face of death only exists on rare occasions. That's the bad news: death shatters all peace of mind. And with mind's peace shattered, so is the ego. That may be the good news and the reason why death can be our most valuable ally. Death forces us out of our minds, our ego-centered minds.

In the face of death, the only possible peace exists outside of the mind, out and beyond the mind's clinging to and fighting for survival. The only peace that can be is the peace that according to the gospels is "not of this world," not of this mind.

So death takes us into the heart of the teachings of the Buddha and the heart of the life of Christ. As such, death is indeed an invaluable ally to the soul.

The yoga of courage and compassion can be considered a gift from the sick and dying to the healthy and living. It gathered its strength at the edge of life, where life meets death. It offers its insights and strengths for use in the midst of life itself, in every moment and every season of it. It offers a sword to cut through the clinging and fighting of our minds, and a hammer to break down the walls between ourselves and life such as it is.

It creates a space for peace to be.

The nine chapters that follow each consist of an introductory text and a series of exercises that transmute the words and ideas found here in this introduction into the living reality of our breath, our body, and our daily actions. The exercises have been carefully selected to explore step-by-step the space beyond the mind, the space of life such as it is. Each chapter builds on the previous chapter, so it is important to first become familiar with the exercises in one chapter before going on to the next.

Your journey begins now, starting with your breath, your breathing out . . .

PART 1

· · · · · · ·

BREATH

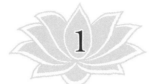

Breathing Out
Letting Yourself Go

A yoga of courage and compassion is not a set of exercises to relax the body and ease the mind. It's more like an adventurous journey or a pilgrimage, the pilgrimage of a lifetime that can change you profoundly. This pilgrimage is no sightseeing tour. It's an expedition full of hazards and demands, at times seemingly frightening and dangerous, but more often simply exciting and eventful. It also has its uneventful, even boring moments—moments where you wonder why, for heaven's sake, you ever embarked on this trip. In these moments of doubt you are tempted to stop and turn back. And also, there is the fear of reaching the end. What then? Is there anything further? How will it be for me? Will I still be the person I know now?

The most difficult part of this journey is the beginning, and the most difficult step is the first step: leaving all that's familiar and comfortable behind, and embracing discomfort and insecurity as those feelings arise. Even more difficult is abandoning all the broken dreams and unfinished business, as disappointments, frustration, and anger are often stronger ties to the past than satisfaction and happiness.

Do you really want to go on this trip? Is your motivation strong enough to make you go, to keep you going, to go all the way?

What is the motor of your motivation? Are you lured by the promise of something better and more beautiful out there, or are you driven by the discontent and disillusionment of being here? Whatever your basic motivation, going on this pilgrimage means primarily *letting go of yourself.*

Many cancer patients sense the depth of these words better than I do. To them it means letting go of continuously clinging to life and resisting death. It means surrendering, deeply relaxing the fibers of their bodies and souls. The idea of letting go takes them into a foreign land, an empty space beyond hope and despair, yet unexpectedly peaceful, silent, and strangely vast and unfathomable.

Of course, this is a rare experience even among cancer patients. How much rarer it must be for most of us who are in the middle of our lives, far from its edge, with its life-threatening illnesses, or where just plain old age lurks.

Cancer patients have to live near sharp edges, forced to face the hard facts of life and death. Most of us are under the illusion that we live at the comfortable center of life, with our dreams, fantasies, and the many activities we think are so important and urgent. Compared to the hard facts of life and death, these things are rather soft and fluffy. The more we wrap our lives up with such soft, fluffy material, the more secure we feel, safely distanced from life's sharp edges.

But maybe this is exactly the reason why we want to go on a journey full of insecurities, hazards, and demands. It may be because our lives are so heavily cushioned with comforts and securities and stuffed with routines that we can no longer breathe freely. Or maybe we suspect that there must be a place where we can breathe a cleaner and purer air.

Siddhartha Gautama, who later became the Buddha, had these very same reasons for leaving the luxury and comforts of his father's palace. Boredom with the easy life literally drove him up the palace walls. Curiosity made him look over them. Courage made him go past them. He went alone—just one loyal attendant to lead him out. Once outside, he saw some of life's realities for the first time: a sick man, an old man, a dead body. They provided him with the hard facts that made him think, grow up, and eventually wake up to real life—life *and* death, total impermanence. It was a mind-blowing experience for this young man who before this had lived the sheltered life of a prince. Now he realized how ephemeral that life was and how he was surrounded by a sea of troubles and suffering. He saw how artificial the walls were that his father had built to keep the real world out. He understood that he had never been in touch with life, because he had never been in touch with death.

The first steps on our trip are very much like Siddhartha's first steps beyond the walls of his father's court. Once outside these walls we will hit the same hard realities that hit Siddhartha, and like him we may also wake up.

After Siddhartha became the Buddha, the Awakened One, he advised others to use the hard fact of death as a most valuable ally for confronting the ego-centered mind. He regarded meditating on death as the most basic and effective of all meditations.

It is said in the Mahaparinirvana Sutra:

> *Of all the footprints*
> *Those of the elephant are supreme.*
> *Similarly, of all mindfulness meditations*
> *Those on death are supreme.*

So we should think and feel like terminally ill cancer patients! As a help to this meditation it is recommended that we follow this simple exercise: attend to the coming and going of the breath. Attending to the breath in this very simple way helps us get to the most direct and intimate knowledge of the basic fact of life: its fleeting and impermanent nature.

How different this is from the basic idea with which Descartes, the father of modern Western philosophy, tried to give himself a foothold in reality: *Cogito, ergo sum,* "I think, therefore I am." The Buddha would probably have said: "I breathe, therefore I am . . . not for very long." *Respiro, ergo non sum.*

Breathing Out

. . . .

🧘 Buddha's Basic Breathing Meditation

And how does someone remain focused on the body in and of itself? Breathing in long, he is aware, "I am breathing in long"; or breathing out long, he is aware, "I am breathing out long." Or breathing in short, he is aware, "I am breathing in short"; or breathing out short, he is aware, "I am breathing out short." He trains himself, "I will breathe in sensitive to the entire body"; he trains himself, "I will breathe out sensitive to the entire body."

SATIPATTHANA SUTTA

The breathing meditation that the Buddha taught is the most effective means to extract the mind from its constant preoccupation with thoughts and emotions. The ordinary functioning mind is totally imprisoned by its thoughts about the future and the past and by its emotions about future and past events. These emotions basically revolve around liking or disliking what happened or is going to be. They can easily develop into intense cravings or deep aversions.

Focusing the attention on the breath means disentangling the mind from past and future events. It helps to bring the mind back to the present moment. This is often called "bringing the mind home."

Focusing the attention on the breath disentangles the mind from myriad emotional reactions ranging from subtle likes and dislikes to the strongest cravings and aversions. This helps create a balanced, tranquil mind. This is called "the tranquil abiding mind."

Focusing the attention on the breath gives us a direct experience of the nature of life and all reality: fleeting and ever changing. Impermanent! Everything that seems solid dissolves and disappears. Matter dissolves into energy.

Focusing the attention on the breath teaches you how to deal with life and its ever-changing nature. Let it go, let it flow, let it happen.

Finally, the breath connects you with the breath of the universe. It connects your mind with universal mind.

◄■►

You can do this breathing meditation in any position you feel comfortable in.

Observe and follow your breath. Feel how the air flows through your nostrils when you breathe in, and how it flows out again when you breathe out.

Do this ten times. Start counting all over again when you realize your mind has completely wandered off.

🧘 Meditative Breathing Exercises

The following exercises will allow for a deepening of the exhalation to happen in a natural way. The first exercise uses some simple movements; the second exercise uses sound; and the third uses a visualization.

Take time to experiment with each one of them and discover for yourself which one has the clearest effect for you.

✻ Breath-Body Movement

Lie down comfortably on your back. Take care that you will not be disturbed, especially by your cell phone.

Focus your attention on your outbreath, and observe how you exhale without changing your breathing pattern in any way. Don't make your outbreath longer, smoother, or quieter because you think that's the way it ought to be. Accept the way you breathe out exactly as it happens at this moment . . .

You will probably notice that just observing the flow of your breathing as it is, not interfering with it, is very difficult, as difficult as accepting yourself just as you are. But you might observe some subtle change, which happens spontaneously.

🌸 After you have done this for a minute or so, slowly breathe in and quietly tense the muscles of both your feet by curling your toes down.

Figure 1.1. Tense the muscles of your feet by curling your toes down.

Hold your breath for a brief moment and then slowly breathe out, relaxing the muscles of your feet completely.

Repeat five times . . .

Relax a minute and observe all the subtle changes and sensations that you experience in your feet and legs.

🌸 Breathe in and pull the front part of your feet toward you, flexing the joints of your ankles.

Figure 1.2. Pull the front part of your feet toward you, flexing the joints of your ankles.

Hold your breath a moment and then slowly breathe out while you relax your feet and ankles.

Repeat five times . . .

Relax and observe attentively all the fleeting sensations in your feet and legs.

🌸 Breathe in and shift your right foot toward you, bending your knee. Hold your breath a moment and then breathe out while simultaneously letting your leg slide down to the floor, relaxing it completely.

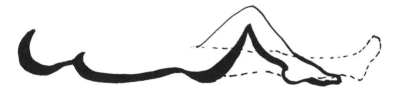

Figure 1.3. Bend your right knee with your inhalation; slide it to the floor when you exhale.

Repeat five times . . .

Do the same with your left foot.

Take a few moments to relax and observe the changes in the way you now breathe. Is your exhalation longer, smoother, and easier? It probably is.

✳ Sound

Lie down comfortably on your back.

Slowly breathe in, and when you breathe out let the sound *HUUU* resonate through your body. Let the sound move through your body, down your legs, and out your feet.

Let the sound dissolve in the open space beneath your feet in the same way a river dissolves in the vastness of the ocean.

Imagine that at the same time all your physical, emotional, and mental tensions dissolve in space.

Repeat five times . . .

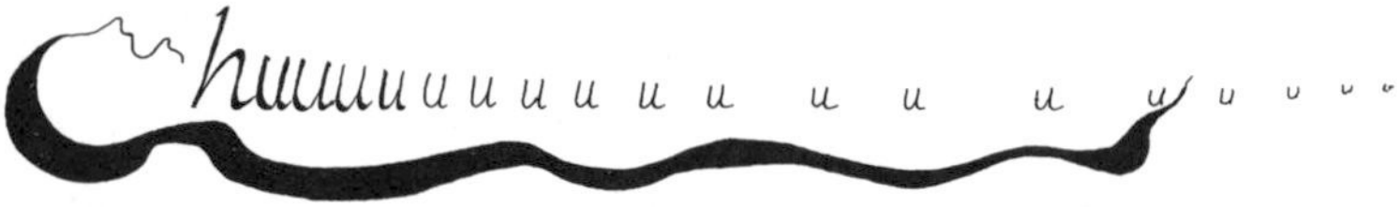

Figure 1.4. As you breathe out, let the sound HUUU resonate through your body.

Relax and observe the changing sensations within and around your body.

✳ Visualization

Imagine that you are lying in the warm golden sand of a quiet beach. In front of you is the wide expanse of a calm ocean. There is hardly any wind.

Right beneath your feet and just above the horizon of the ocean, visualize the sun as a magnificent golden-orange orb.

Breathe in and let your whole body be filled with the pure, healthy air of the ocean.

Hold your breath a moment, and then slowly breathe out and let your breath slowly flow down and out of your body just like the *HUUU* sound in the previous exercise. Visualize your breath as a river flowing down your body and out into the ocean and on toward that magnificent sun beneath your feet.

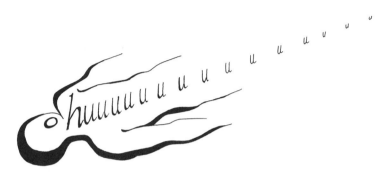

Figure 1.5. Visualize your breath as a river flowing down your body, out into the ocean, and on toward a magnificent sun beneath your feet.

Imagine that the radiance of this sun grows as your breath reaches and enters it.

Repeat five times . . .

As you identify more and more with your breath, you may be able to let yourself go in the exhalation, disconnecting from your tight mind-set and disturbing thoughts and emotions. Left to themselves, they are deflated and powerless.

Relax, observe, and enjoy the open, free, and clear feeling.

🧘 Back to Buddha's Basic Breathing Meditation

Again try to follow ten cycles of your natural breathing with full attention.

You may discover a definite change in your breathing pattern from the first time you did this meditation. The previous exercises may have changed the quality and depth of your exhalation, but when one element is changed, the whole is changed. This is just as true for the breath as it is for a family, a society, or for global ecology.

◄■►

Don't get discouraged when you find out how difficult it is to keep your attention on your breath. Actually, one of the normal effects of this exercise is that you will discover how easily distracted, busy, and unruly your mind is, or how stubborn and lazy. Don't think that it's just you who has this problem or that you aren't the right kind of person for this type of thing. This is exactly how the ordinary mind functions, mine and yours. It shows how very little we are in control of our minds. We need this discovery to strengthen our motivation to master our minds and free them from the merry-go-round of constant thinking and conflicting emotions.

Congratulate yourself for the very short moments— maybe seconds—that you managed to keep your mind focused on your breath. Collect these seconds as if they were precious grains of gold.

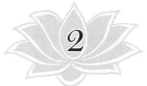

Breathing Pause
Venturing Emptiness

Once you've conquered your fears, thus allowing you to let go of the familiar and the comfortable, you start on your pilgrimage, this yoga of courage and compassion. A new world opens for you. Once you've stepped out of the courtyard of your father's palace, you look into a dazzling, wide-open space in front of you and all around you. It's the open space of the real world, full of its strange and unfamiliar sounds and smells, sights and colors.

After all those months and maybe years of delaying your departure and holding on to the duties and responsibilities of daily life, there is now this wonderful, exhilarating feeling of freedom. You realize you've done it! You've taken your first step. You finally have the courage to go. And to your great relief, you discover that you do not fall into a black hole. Your feet actually meet the solid ground of the earth. You discover that there is a real world out there, and that you can safely breathe in the air of its free and open space. All your former fears and fantasies of stepping outside and plunging into some dark abyss of utter emptiness subside.

The haze that covers everything and envelops your whole being has just lifted. You realize how the business of your own ordinary life has created it. You have lived in a multitude of daily worries and anxieties, a turmoil of constant thoughts and emotions that coalesce into an enveloping opaque cloud. You realize that this is exactly the reason why you so badly need to leave. You started to feel claustrophobic inside your very own life. You simply were not happy.

You take your first step and inadvertently let out a big sigh of relief—the relief of finally having broken away from it all and surviving. Breath is here again. It just released itself. Like a bird set free, it spreads its wings. This very sigh of relief is "breathing out" and flying into the wide open space of the world all around you. This exhalation compels you to venture further into this new, free world.

The breath is your only guide and companion. Like Siddhartha leaving his father's court, you have in your breath a loyal servant to lead the way, away from all the tenacious clinging to the secure and familiar—your house, your friends, your possessions, your old ways of thinking, feeling, and behaving. In your first big sigh of relief you start to let go of these tensions. You relax.

So this pilgrimage is already different from what you had imagined it to be. You thought you would tumble into a no-man's-land, but instead you find yourself in an open space where all the sights and sounds appear much clearer and nearer. Now nothing seems to separate you from your surroundings. Nothing fogs up your senses. There is so much to see, hear, and smell! When you left home you feared poverty, but instead you find the abundant richness of the real world, a richness filled with life and death, birthing and dying.

Are there limits to your fully experiencing and enjoying all this abundance? Not if your senses and heart stay open and you do not cling to anything or anybody for as long as you are on this trip.

You may go anywhere, but you are never allowed to stay.

You can meet all sorts of people, even fall in love with some of them, but you are never allowed to become attached.

You may enjoy everything, but without possessing.

You are not allowed to keep anything that you receive. You have to part with it right away, giving away what you do not really need and emptying your pockets before moving on.

This pilgrimage is about learning to give. Giving is regarded as the first virtue to be mastered on the path to enlightenment. Buddhists call this the *first paramita*.

Again the breath is your guide and companion. This kind of giving is like breathing out totally and completely, not retaining anything of the last breath. To fully breathe out, you need to become completely empty at each exhalation, completely silent . . .

In many schools of mysticism the empty moment between the outbreath and the inbreath, the breathing pause, is considered crucial. It opens the secret door into a wide, silent inner space . . . To emptiness. Fullness!

The breath as your loyal attendant shows you the secret passage into this empty space, so full of life and death. The breath is your faithful companion and trustworthy guide on this trip. Are you willing to follow this guide? Are you able to follow your breath all the way out?

Probably, like most people, you used to breathe out just halfway, then quickly breathe in again. You did not allow for the empty space, that precious moment of silence between your outbreath and your inbreath. In this way your inbreath could never rise from its true depths. Your breathing pattern thus remained stuck in a cycle of shallow outbreaths and inbreaths, perpetuating the continuous cycle of thoughts and emotions, the product of your ego mind. When you breathed partially like this, you held your breath, thereby forcing it to follow you instead of you following it. But now, when you breathe out fully, it means that you will follow your breath all the way out, venturing past the last outpost of your ego mind.

Attending and following the breath as the Buddha taught is therefore an extremely important meditation. Its simpleness belies its power and impact. It needs much more courage than you thought would be needed because it involves your most basic fear: letting yourself go. It also requires that you exercise a lot of patience and compassion for yourself so you can loosen up and "step into space."

Breathing Pause

🧘 Buddha's Basic Breathing Meditation

Find a comfortable position and follow ten cycles of breathing with full attentiveness.

🧘 Meditative Breathing Exercises

This time we will focus the attention on the breathing pause, the "empty" moment between breathing out and breathing in.

You may have already discovered a change in your breathing pause after having done the exercises in chapter 1. Changing the quality of your exhalation always has some effect on the next moment in the breathing cycle. In this way you will have discovered how changing one element always has a natural effect on other elements, as everything is interdependent with everything else.

The exercises in this chapter will help you create more space in the breathing pause.

As with the exercises in chapter 1, the exercise that follows uses simple movement. The exercise after that uses sound, and the third, visualization. We will conclude these exercises by going back to the Buddha's Basic Breathing Meditation.

◄■►

✸ Breath-Body Movement

Lie down comfortably on your back.

Breathe in and tense the muscles of both your feet, curling

your toes down. At the same time slightly press your heels
into the floor. This creates tension in the muscles of your legs.
Don't overdo it; these exercises are meant to build up awareness rather than muscle.

*Figure 2.1. Tense the muscles of your feet by
curling your toes down.*

Hold the breath for just a second and then slowly release
the tension while you exhale completely, right into that silent,
empty space beyond the last bit of your outbreath. Take care
not to push the last bit of breath out. Let it flow out of you in
a very easy and natural way.

Feel how the sense of relaxation expands from the insides
of your feet and legs outward into the surrounding space.

Do not repeat this exercise right away. Allow yourself to
enjoy the new feeling of relaxation. Let one breathing cycle
(in—out—pause) pass before you do the exercise again.

Repeat three times . . .

🌺 Breathe in and tense the muscles of both your hands,
making fists. At the same time, press your fists against the
floor, creating tension in both your arms.

Hold the breath for a second and then slowly relax your
arms and hands, turning the palms of your hands toward the
floor. Let the breath quietly flow out of you. Feel it flowing
down and out of your arms and hands into the open space

that surrounds them. Enjoy the new feeling of relaxation and the inner silence that comes with it.

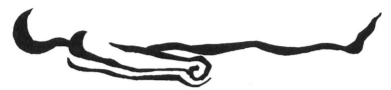

Figure 2.2. Press your fists against the floor, creating tension in both your arms.

Guard this silence.
Let one breathing cycle pass (in—out—pause).
Repeat three times . . .

❀ Breathe in and tense the muscles of your face, at the same time pressing the back of your head lightly against the floor. You will become aware of a tension in the muscles of your back. Hold the breath for a second and then release all this tension while you exhale. Feel the tension disappear in all directions, right through the skin of your head and back.

Figure 2.3. Breathe in and tense the muscles of your face, at the same time pressing the back of your head lightly against the floor.

Guard the silence that is now in and around you while letting a full breathing cycle pass (in—out—pause).
Repeat three times . . .

✳ Sound

In this exercise we combine movement and sound.

◄■►

Lie down comfortably on your back.

Breathe in and tense the muscles of your feet, hands, face, and buttocks.

Hold the breath for a moment and then release the tension while breathing out and making the sound *OOOHH*...

Let the sound disappear in silence...

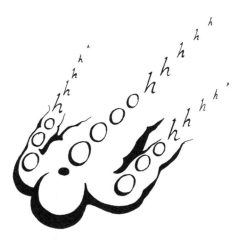

Figure 2.4. Release tension while breathing out and making the sound OOOHH.

Guard this silence while a full breathing cycle revolves within you like a wave in the ocean.

Like the *HUUU* of the previous chapter, this *OOOHH* may release residual mental, emotional, and physical tension, even pain.

Don't think about it or (psycho)analyze it. Just let it happen and let it go.

Repeat three times . . .

❋ Now, without tensing or moving the muscles of your body, slowly breathe in and quietly breathe out with a soundless *OOO*. Imagine that this time your *OOO* is beautifully clear and open (therefore now without the *HH* sound). Use your acoustic imagination. Don't make the sound out loud, but instead hear the sound inside of you.

Let this *OOO* expand outward in increasingly wider circles, right through the skin of your body and into the space surrounding you.

Let the *OOO* dissolve in silence. You may notice that your lips naturally touch each other after you breathe out, forming the silent sound *MMM*. In this way, and without trying, you chanted the holy syllable *OM*.

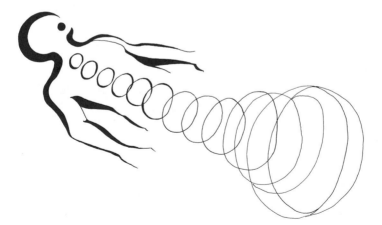

Figure 2.5. Expand the OOO in widening circles around your body, allowing it to naturally close with MMM, creating the holy syllable OM.

Expand the *OOO* in widening circles around your body, allowing it to naturally close with *MMM,* creating the holy syllable *OM.*

Guard this silence and let a whole breathing cycle effortlessly flow through you.

Repeat three times . . .

✳ Visualization

Lie down comfortably on your back.

Breathe in, and while you breathe out, visualize the breath as crystal-clear water flowing down your body and out of you.

Imagine the source of this river is approximately one-and-a-half feet above your head, and visualize this river flowing out into a vast ocean.

Go with the flow . . .

Identify yourself with it and experience that exquisite moment when the river flows beyond the confining boundaries of the riverbed reaching the ocean (see figure 2.6).

Let your mind stay awhile in that vast expanse that is now all around you.

It may help you to stay there a little longer if you silently repeat *OOO . . . MMM* and fill all that space with this sound.

Repeat this three times . . .

✳ Let go of the image of a source, a river, and the ocean. Retain the sense of boundless openness in your mind.

Let this be your experiencing the boundless openness of this present moment, the vast space of the here and now. This space easily encompasses and accommodates everything that

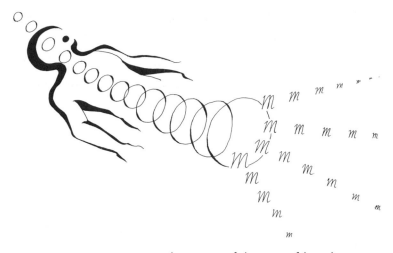

Figure 2.6. Imagine the source of the river of breath approximately one-and-a-half feet above your head, and visualize this river flowing out into a vast ocean.

surrounds you: the furniture in your room, your house, your street, your city, your country, and all people. You don't need to shrink back from them to keep your quiet. On the other hand you should not allow these things and all those people to clog up your mind; otherwise the sense of space is lost.

Guard your mind's space and welcome reality around and within you. Experience how boundless space and the diversity of concrete reality go hand in hand.

🧘 Back to Buddha's Basic Breathing Meditation

Empty your mind of all the previous exercises, images, and words. Come back to the basic breathing meditation.

Follow ten cycles of breathing with full attentiveness.

Maybe you are able to remain completely focused on your breath for a few seconds. Congratulate yourself for it, this might be your first glimpse of nirvana! But don't crave more, as this craving is your most serious trap. It's more important to discover and appreciate the impermanence of these moments of nirvana.

Breathing In

Allowing Life Back In Again

You are out in the open now, breathing freely in the bountiful space of this wide world. Your own breath sets you free. You enjoy the good feeling of having finally been able to let yourself go. It required a lot of courage to take this step, and you will need a lot more courage to continue. The world you just stepped into may be a wonderful space, full of sound and color, but it is not a place you can walk around in with eyes closed and a blissful smile on your face. It is not a quiet suburban park, but nevertheless it is a very real world. You have to watch out not to bump against a car or step in dog shit. There are planes to catch, luggage to guard, and money to change. There are hundreds of people who make a living out of you. You are surrounded by millions of people who stay home, still very much occupied with making their places more secure and comfortable, worrying about their families' future, feeding their bank accounts, being respectable citizens. They are not at all interested in you and your pilgrimage. They smile at you as long as they expect goodies from you.

Once you are shocked into seeing this reality, it's hard to hold on to your newfound peace. You have lots of good reasons to become distrustful of everything and everybody. It's even difficult not to become a bit paranoid, seeing adversaries and enemies all around you. Your newfound world is not just full of beautiful colors and sounds, but also full of all the old familiar egos.

It is into this world that you have stepped.

The big challenge is to see this world clearly, yet without getting entangled in it. The moment you get entangled in it and start to fight it or resist it, the sense of spaciousness is lost. In a flash you would be back where you came from. You might have found a momentary solution to your paranoia, but you will suffer an even nastier bout of anxiety if you get entangled in this kind of world again.

So the challenge is to see all this clearly, and yet trust the space you just stepped into and keep your heart open to this world. Again, this requires courage, but also a great deal of compassion for those people who are not pilgrims. As a result, you have arrived at a new place where you recognize the futility of grasping, fighting, and resisting, realizing that there is much more to life than all that money-mindedness.

And suddenly your wave of paranoia subsides and you let yourself sink even deeper into the wide open spaces of this world. You do not worry about what can be taken away from you. You relax, and again you are open to all the sounds and colors around you. So much more comes to you than can possibly be taken away from you.

And you breathe in . . . a full, deep breath. This breath comes out of the very depths of the wide-open space you just stepped into. You do not "take" this breath. Taking is part of the old life you just gave up. This breath you *receive*. Receiving is a very important principle you have to learn to cultivate in this new life. It is an art to be learned patiently and diligently upon every inbreath. Inhaling in this way can be an exhilarating and joyful discovery. Graceful . . . blissful . . . the unexpected reward for having had the courage to go on this pilgrimage.

If you followed your outbreath, who is now following your inbreath? Is it the same old you returning to your old premises, or does someone or something new come in? Life? Death? Bliss?

Questions arise: Are you arriving at the end of the journey, or is the end of the journey arriving at you? Where does the destination of this pilgrimage lie? Somewhere out there, or right here?

The pilgrimage of a lifetime—beginning it, traveling it, arriving at the final destination—seems to happen in one cycle of breath.

Breathing In
· ·

🧘 *Buddha's Basic Breathing Meditation*

Find a comfortable position and follow ten cycles of breathing with full attentiveness.

🧘 *Meditative Breathing Exercises*

The focus of your attention will now be your inbreath.

The following exercises may help you to allow the inbreath to happen by itself. You will recognize elements from the previous exercises.

◄■►

Allow yourself a few moments to observe how you breathe in. Notice whether you "take" a breath or whether you really allow your breath to come in by itself, welcoming it. Try to observe yourself and your way of breathing honestly. Remember that any change you deliberately create in your breathing pattern will inevitably lead to a "taking" of the breath. Don't get disheartened if you observe that you're doing exactly that. Smile, relax, and breathe again.

✳ Breath-Body Movement

Lie down comfortably on your back.

Breathe in and wrap both of your hands around your right knee, drawing it in toward your chest (see figure 3.1). Do not let your breath be pushed up too much into your chest, but let it find extra space in your left and right side,

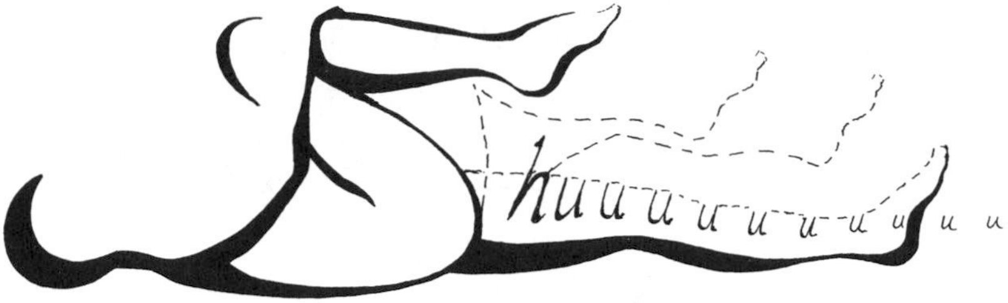

Figure 3.1. Hug your right knee, drawing it toward your chest.

your lower back, and even the bottom of your pelvis.

Hold your breath a moment and then slide your leg down while you breathe out with the silent sound *HUUU*.

Let your breath dissolve in the space beneath your feet. Let the sound dissolve in silence.

Guard this silence during one full cycle of breathing.

Repeat three times . . .

Do the same movement with your left leg.

✳ Sound

Lie down flat on your back with both legs comfortably resting on the floor and your feet approximately one-and-a-half feet apart.

Breathe in, and when you breathe out let the sound *HUUMMM* travel down your body like water through a river to finally flow out into a wide-open sea. The moment the sound leaves your body it changes from *HUUU* into *MMM* . . . (See figure 3.2 on page 34.)

Imagine that this *MMM* fills the entire sea.

Repeat three times . . .

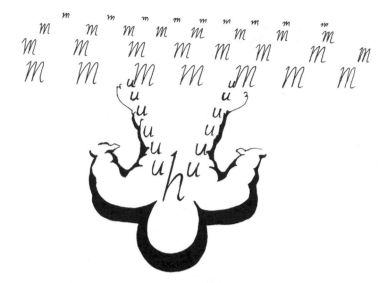

Figure 3.2. Let the sound HUUMMM *travel down
your body like a river and beyond, out into a wide-open sea.*

🪷 After the third time take a moment to relax and discover how the *MMM* sound created a subtle vibration between and around your lips. Feel how this vibration deeply relaxes your lips and face. You may find yourself smiling a bit. If so, let this smile spread over your face, throat, and chest, and over your entire body.

Experience the spreading of this smile and the sweet joy this brings. Body and mind are now so deeply relaxed that all the business, all the wanting, needing, and desiring are gone.

You are at peace with yourself.

There is no need to "take" the next breath. It will come by itself. You receive it.

Allow yourself to deeply enjoy this receiving of the breath. Let it fill you completely.

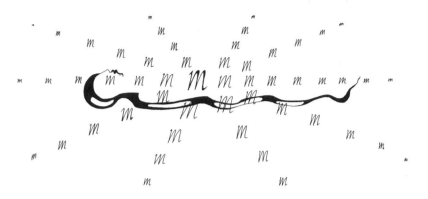

Figure 3.3. Experience the resonance of MMM on your lips and the resulting smile and peace spreading over your entire body.

Somewhere in the depths of your soul the *MMM* still resonates. In the *MMM* there is deep joy, gratefulness, bliss . . .

✳ Visualization

Let go of the images of river and sea. You don't need them anymore. With these images gone, try now to maintain a sense of boundless openness. This boundless openness is the mind's basic quality beyond all thoughts and emotions.

Experience the boundless space of the present moment, the here and now. The space of your mind and the space of this moment are fundamentally one and the same.

This space easily encompasses and accommodates all of reality surrounding you. Everything around you at this very moment is part of your here and now.

Imagine that when you breathe in you receive all the good qualities and energies that surround you—from the earth beneath you, heaven above you, and nature all around you.

Imagine that you also receive the positive energies of millions of people around the globe and throughout the ages, all their selfless thoughts and prayers.

Conclude this exercise with the following sequence of sounds:

OM . . . (breathing in)

AH . . . (holding the breath)

HUM . . . (breathing out)

With the *HUM* visualize yourself radiating positive energy out in all directions. Now it is you who gives out boundless positive energy selflessly.

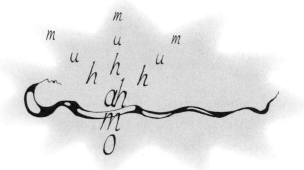

Figure 3.4. Radiate positive energy in all directions.

🧘 Back to Buddha's Basic Breathing Meditation

Follow ten cycles of breathing with focused attention. If you discover that concentrating on ten breathing cycles is too many, try two sets of five cycles.

PART 2

BREATH
AND BODY

4

The Pelvic Bowl
Accepting with Compassion

This entire pilgrimage has turned out to be about going nowhere in particular, going to no specific place, in no foreign country, in no strange world. There is no holy shrine to visit, no holy man to meet, no special destination to reach.

This pilgrimage is about stepping into the reality of this world, as painful and beautiful as it is. And this world—this real world—is everywhere around you, right here and now. You need cross no distance, purchase no ticket.

This pilgrimage is about stepping into the depth of space. It is more vertical than horizontal. It takes you inside rather than outside. It takes you into a vast, wide-open space in which the horizontal and the vertical, the inside and the outside, the painful and the joyful are all encompassed.

In this space there is no contradiction between in or out, up or down, here or there. You step into the reality of One. Actually, what you left behind is the confusion of two, of living in two worlds, a real one and an idealized one. Exactly this confusion of being two—and often many more!—fogged up your mind so much that you ended up living in a cloud, the cloud of a constantly disturbed mind with all its contradictory emotions, its likes and dislikes, its desires and aversions. All these dualities kept you ensnared in a multitude of alternatives and choices.

According to Buddhism living in this cloud means living in ego-created samsara. The worst is that we aren't even aware of it! Buddhists call this lack of awareness *ignorance*.

So the step you took basically takes you out of your mind, out of your disturbed and confused ego.

At this moment you may not be aware of the far-reaching implications of this step. You actually step out of your mind and into your body. This is not the body you see in the mirror, about which you always had mixed feelings and critical judgments. This body in the mirror is caught in the claws of your ego mind or, more gently put, shrouded in a cloud of ignorance.

Few people are able to look at themselves with an open, nonjudgmental mind and with kind and compassionate eyes. They always think they should be thinner, stronger, more beautiful, or better exercised. Somehow, that mirrored body always falls short of the standards of beauty and youth they carry in their heads. We are always measuring the distance between our real bodies and our idealizations, judging what is good and what is bad about it, thereby continually creating splits, the body-mind split above all.

But our body is exactly as good or bad as it is. Its plain and sober truth is that it is as it is, tall or short, thin or heavy, young or old. Inevitably it starts to wrinkle, bend, and sag, eventually to wither and die. Rather brutally, our bodies confront our ego minds with the Buddha's First Noble Truth: the truth of our life's impermanence and the suffering that necessarily comes from not accepting that.

If you allow yourself to step into your body with your mind unclouded by judgments, then you are actually stepping into the naked reality of physical existence. You step into a free and open space beyond all your judgments and conflicting emotions. You step right through that layer of fantasy and illusion that our minds constantly wrap around this basic reality. Like Alice in Wonderland, you step through the looking glass into a very different world, only this world is not a fairy tale—it is very real!

In taking this step you abandon your mind's continuous obsession about your body's appearance and health, letting go of your mental clouds of judgments, emotions, and wishful thinking. When those clouds disappear, your real body appears, and you can at last fully experience it with all your senses. You will then become truly sensuous and sensitive.

You may also discover that most of your physical tensions disappear at the same time, as those clouds did not simply hang around the body but also entered your skin and penetrated deep into the fibers of your muscles and organs. Those mental clouds are the stuff of stress and physical tension. Only when you let go of these clouds will you be able to really relax.

And if you are relaxed you can now honestly face yourself as you are and face reality as it is. You hit, as it were, rock bottom, the essential core of things. It may be your first hard awakening to the truth of life, similar to how it was for Siddhartha when he left his father's palace. Apparently, a hard awakening is first needed to eventually attain enlightenment.

So your pilgrimage does not take you into some foreign country. It launches you into the depths of reality, which also means the depths of your body. This word *depth* has to be understood in a very literal sense. It means the bottom of your pelvis, through your legs, to the soles of your feet. Breathing out into the very depth of your body, you may discover that you do not fall into a hole, but into a "bowl"—the bowl of your pelvis.

This kind of breathing is so far out that it requires letting go of the ego. Letting go of the ego always means facing our fear of death. Not fearing death is so far out that it may seem impossible, as impossible as it was for that camel in the gospel having to go through the eye of a needle.

And even if that camel could have managed to get through, what would have become of him? How much camel would have been left of him when he arrived on the other side? The paradoxical truth is that only the camel that is able to let himself go will find his passage through the needle's eye.

It is evident that the camel that Christ talked about is the camel of our ego. This ego has to go—has to die—if we are to enter that all-encompassing space on the other side of the needle's eye.

The eye of the needle may be found right in the heart of death, the ego's death. It is right through this eye—the death of the I—that the kingdom of heaven can be found:

the dazzling, all-encompassing, and infinitely compassionate space of reality itself. It totally accepts and welcomes you exactly as you are, without all the fantasies of who you would like to be.

You can leave everything that is not truly you behind. You can unburden yourself and finally relax.

The Pelvic Bowl

🧘 Buddha's Basic Breathing Meditation

Find a comfortable position and follow ten cycles of breathing with full attentiveness.

🧘 Meditative Breathing Exercises

The exercises in this chapter help you get more grounded in the depth of your pelvic floor. This can radically alter your sense of self, as you are no longer experiencing yourself from your head down, with all the judgments and self-criticism that you bring in from there.

◄■►

✹ Breath-Body Movement

Sit straight but relaxed in a chair or, if you are comfortable with it, in a cross-legged or half-lotus position on a cushion on the floor.

Try to feel how your sitting bones touch the surface of the seat of your chair or cushion.

Roll over them by tilting your pelvis forward and backward. This movement should be in the lower half of your body; the upper half of your body should remain as still as possible. Observe when you inhale and exhale. Move gently backward and forward in the natural rhythm of your breathing (see figure 4.1 on page 44).

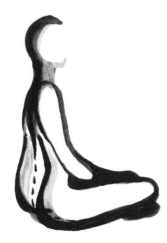

Figure 4.1. Tilt the pelvis forward and backward to the natural rhythm of your breathing.

Repeat ten times . . .

Pause awhile and observe your breath and other sensations in your body without interfering.

❀ Stretch your spine a bit and rotate it in its full length, five times to the right and, after a short pause, five times to the left (see figure 4.2).

Pause and observe your breath and other sensations throughout your body.

❀ Slowly bend your head forward while you relax all the muscles in your face. Let a few breathing cycles pass by. Slowly raise your head (see figure 4.3).

Repeat three times . . .

Pause and observe your breath and other sensations throughout your body. Observe how they arise and disappear of their own accord.

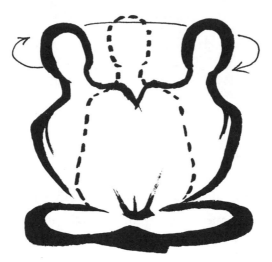

Figure 4.2. Rotate your spine five times
in each direction.

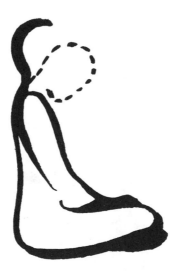

Figure 4.3. Slowly bend your head forward while you
relax all the muscles in your face.

✳ Sound and Visualization

Sit straight but relaxed in a chair or, if you are comfortable with it, in a cross-legged or half-lotus position on a cushion on the floor.

Feel your two sitting bones. Imagine how they root themselves deeper into the floor or in the seat of your chair. It helps to visualize this in a warm orange color.

Do the same with your tailbone.

The sitting bones and tailbone together form a triangle that firmly connects you right through the pelvic floor to the earth beneath. At the same time keep your legs and feet relaxed and well connected to your pelvis.

Notice whether this triangle helps you sink deeper

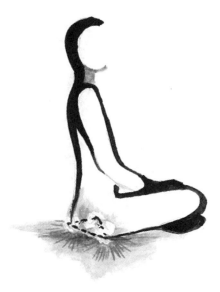

Figure 4.4. The sitting bones and tailbone together form a triangle that firmly connects you right through the pelvic floor to the earth beneath.

into the pelvis, with a deeper sense of connectedness to the earth.

Does this also subtly change the way you breathe?

✻ Let the sound *HUUU* resonate in the space of your pelvis. Experiment with whether it is more effective to make the sound aloud or silently.

Imagine that your pelvis becomes deeper, rounder, and wider while you are doing this and how it gradually assumes the form of a beautiful shining bowl.

See it as an energy form, a creation of your own mind. It is therefore not opaque and heavy, but transparent and light, open to the earth beneath you and toward you.

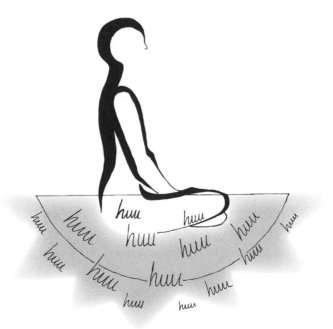

Figure 4.5. Allow the energy of your pelvis to form a beautiful shining bowl.

You may experience this bowl even more clearly when you circle your attention through it. Circle three times clockwise, to the right, and three times counterclockwise.

Now, stop making the sound and take a few moments to experience this bowl. Do you feel comfortable in it and supported by it?

How does it change the way you breathe?

✳ Visualization and Beyond

Visualizing this bowl is a tremendous help in creating the experience of encompassing, all-embracing space within and around you. This encompassing space is not just a mental abstraction but a real experience that can be felt throughout your body.

Experiencing yourself from the bottom of this bowl upward is markedly different from experiencing yourself from the head downward. From the head there is always critical thinking and judgment. From the bowl upward you can experience profound and nonjudgmental self-acceptance, true compassion for yourself.

◄■►

Sit quietly for five minutes and observe yourself in a friendly and compassionate way. Remember to smile!

Observe especially all the physical and emotional sensations in and throughout your body. Observe how they continuously change while keeping your awareness on them.

In doing this you discover firsthand that none of these sensations are fixed and permanent. Everything in your body, like everything in life, is in a constant state of flux.

With the aid of this bowl you can very accurately observe all the changes that take place. It's like watching a river flowing by or the constantly changing clouds in the sky.

🧘 Adapting Buddha's Basic Breathing Meditation

Now we introduce a change in this meditation.

◄■►

Instead of observing the flow of your breath through your nostrils, imagine that pure cosmic energy enters the space of your pelvic bowl right through your sacrum, the large triangular bone at the base of the spine, in the back of the pelvis. Don't think of your pelvis as something compact and impenetrable, but instead imagine it to be transparent and permeable.

5

The Spinal Column
Courageously Facing Reality

When the ego mind looks at itself in the mirror, it never sees its true and real face. Less and less in touch with reality, it always sees its own projections. It is increasingly isolated and lonely. True consciousness—consciousness beyond the ego mind—is like the mirror itself, reflecting reality honestly and exactly. It observes everything—life and death, courage and cowardice, in short, all that is. Mental acrobatics cannot discover this consciousness; however, a jump out of the mind's acrobatics and a dive into the depths of our body's space can and will.

One discovers consciousness beyond ego mind by venturing beyond the mental constrictions in one's head and beyond the web of emotions around one's heart. Pure consciousness manifests itself when the space of the pelvis is open, relaxed, and well connected with the earth beneath and the world around. The restricted anatomical form of the pelvis then transforms into a wide, large, round bowl. This bowl shines like a beautifully polished mirror, reflecting every detail of

one's being—physical, emotional, and mental—in an abso-
lutely nonjudgmental and very compassionate way.

This quality of consciousness can only manifest after the
outbreath has entered the bowl of the pelvis, a precinct that
is sacred and at the same time very down-to-earth. Then one
can say that the breath has entered the metaphorical kingdom
of heaven after having gone through the eye of the needle. In
the process mind as we know it has gone. It has died.

At this point Buddhists say that one has become a tatha-
gata, one gone beyond, gone beyond the cloud of ignorance
that created a safe distance between oneself and reality as it is.
All suffering basically arises out of this distance that chains
us in the restless merry-go-round of samsara. This suffering
has been every pilgrim's motivation for leaving worldly life
and going on pilgrimage.

Crossing this distance always requires stopping the igno-
rant mind by cutting through the dualistic thinking that
gives rise to the basic passions of desire and anger: the desire
to cling to the pleasurable, and anger at whatever thwarts the
fulfillment of desire.

A mind that is clear, untainted by passions and drives,
could be called a "virginal" mind. It is open, free of likes and
dislikes, and receptive.

Having a virginal mind has nothing to do with being
prudish or never having had sex. It also has nothing to do
with being a woman or a man. It means experiencing something as if it were happening for the very first time, be it sex,
a sunset, or a glass of wine. There is no comparing with previous experiences or anticipating future ones.

Only with a virginal mind can one conceive consciousness

beyond ego mind. Only as such a virgin can one give birth to the untainted, immaculate consciousness of the true essence of reality. Only through one's outbreath into the womb of the body can one father it.

After having conceived this immaculate consciousness, your breath has to closely and diligently guard and nourish it as though it were a fetus in your womb. The full cycle of your breathing—the outbreath, the silence, the inbreath—needs to move in the open space of your pelvis, revolving around and within its center. This requires undivided attention and mindfulness beyond the dualistic mind: a mind that is virginal, motherly, still.

Then, after some time, something will happen in the center of your mind and the inner space of your pelvis, your energetic or literal womb: you will feel an energy, an inner warmth, a sense of subtle, exquisite life. This is *chi,* or *qi.*

At times it is visible to the inner eye as a light. Then one can understand why in different spiritual traditions consciousness has been equated with light, and why the awakening of consciousness has been described as "the dawning of light," as in Buddha's enlightenment or Christ's birth as the coming of the light into the world.

After this light is born in the center of your mind and womb, it will gain strength and will rise up the spine, vertebra after vertebra. It can really be experienced as a subtle energy that fills the whole spinal column, cleansing and strengthening the nerve centers on its way. This creates a very definite and often glorious feeling of lightness and transparency, inner strength, self-confidence, and an unmistakable courage to be.

In Tibetan Buddhism a very similar experience is called

"arising as a deity," when a divine quality manifests in and through our human body. In Christianity it can be regarded as the Resurrection of Jesus Christ, not signifying the physical resurrection of his body out of the grave two thousand years ago, but the arising of our own immaculate Christ consciousness in our body and mind, here and now.

The truth is that the pivotal spiritual events of the great religions of the world are not far-out stories about extraordinary people in distant times and places. No, they are about us and about our innermost, most intimate experiences. There is actually no distance between the essence of our own spiritual experience and those crucial events of 2,000 and 2,600 years ago. In reality there is no distance between our innermost being and the Christ and the Buddha. The courage that is ultimately required of us is the courage to annihilate this distance. The moment this distance is destroyed there will no longer be a worshipper, a worshipped one, or worshipping— only the one Self, the one Buddha, the one Christ. All One.

If giving birth to the light and the resurrection of the light are fundamentally one and the same thing, then the distance between Christmas and Easter is dissolved. Thus the bridge from Christmas to Easter may be the ever-stronger realization of the light through the phases of a woman's or man's life, including through the phase of physical death.

As the body is the metaphorical temple of Jerusalem, we are first destroyed so that we may be rebuilt from the ground up: from the base of the pelvis, up the spine, to the crown of the head, and beyond.

That is the reason to meditate, solidly grounded in the earth and with an erect spine. Then the light you birth finds its way through you—through your body, your mind, and throughout all of your life. It opens you and connects you to the earth below and heaven above. It opens you to life *and* death, dissolving your clinging to life and your fearing death. It opens your heart to loving-kindness. It clears your mind so you can see the One in all, or God in everything as Christians say, and realizing the emptiness of all phenomena, as Buddhists say.

The Spinal Column

🧘 Buddha's Basic Breathing Meditation

Find a comfortable position and follow ten cycles of breathing with full attentiveness.

🧘 Meditative Breathing Exercises

Breathe in through your sacrum and let the breath fill the empty sacred space in the middle of your pelvic bowl.

Observe how the breath gathers vitalizing cosmic energy within this most special and intimate place in your body.

Keep your mind focused in this area and notice any change that happens there. Don't will or fantasize anything. Receive graciously whatever happens with an open and pure mind.

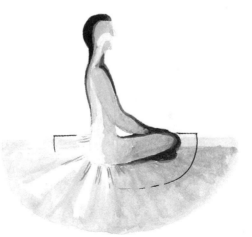

Figure 5.1. Breathe in through your sacrum into the empty sacred space in the middle of your pelvic bowl.

✳ Breath-Body Movement

Sit straight in a chair or cross-legged or in half-lotus on a cushion on the floor.

Connect with the earth beneath you through the triangle formed by your two sitting bones and your tailbone.

Then try to stretch your spinal column by simultaneously pushing your tailbone deeper into the floor and extending the back of your head upward toward the sky while keeping your chin tucked in.

Let the breath come and go.

Release the stretch, leaving a sense of extension in the spine.

Repeat three times . . .

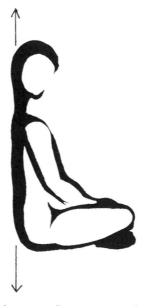

Figure 5.2. Push your tailbone into the floor and extend the back of your head upward toward the sky.

❧ Twist your spine along its axis to the left. Use your hands to support you, pushing with your right hand against the inside of your right knee and placing your left hand on the floor behind your back. If you're sitting on a chair, you can grab a side or the back of your chair as a support.

Turn your head over your shoulder to the left and look backward. Retain that extended feeling along your spine.

Relax the rest of your body as much as possible as you twist, keeping your shoulders low.

Let the breath come and go a couple of times in a relaxed and natural way.

Turn slowly back to the normal position and do the same movement to the right side, turning your head to the right and looking backward.

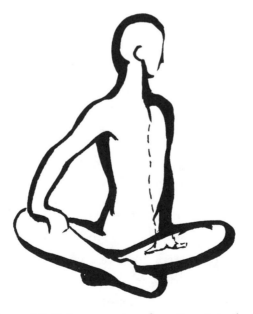

Figure 5.3. Twist your spine along its axis to the left.

Repeat once again in both directions.

Observe the breath and the flow of sensations in your body.

🌺 Slowly bend your head forward. Relax all the muscles in your face. Feel the stretch all the way down your back.

Let the breath come and go naturally . . .

Raise your head to an upright position and experience again that extended feeling along your spine from your coccyx up to the back of your head and beyond . . .

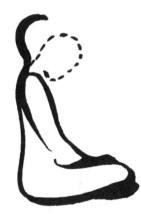

Figure 5.4. Slowly bend your head forward and relax all the muscles in your face.

Repeat this three times . . .

🌺 Following these three exercises take a few moments to sit still and relax. Remember the bowl in and around your pelvis.

Experience the energy form of that bowl together with the straight line of your spine.

Experience the combination of a sense of roundness and straightness in and through your body.

Observe your breath and the flow of physical and emotional sensations in a relaxed, detached manner.

✳ Sound

Sit straight in a chair or cross-legged or in half-lotus on a cushion on the floor.

Slowly breathe in, and when you breathe out let the sound *HUUU* travel down your spine. Direct this sound right through the empty space in the middle of your pelvic bowl in front of your sacrum and then down to the bottom of your bowl.

Imagine this bottom to be one-and-a-half feet beneath your pelvic floor.

The moment you reach the bottom of your bowl, the sound *HUUU* changes into *MMM . . .*

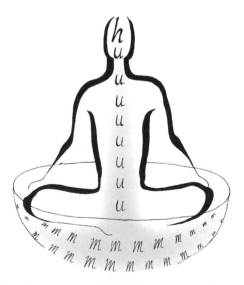

Figure 5.5. Breathe the sound HUUU *down your spine and down the empty space in the middle of your pelvic bowl to its very bottom.*

In doing this you're making the sound *HUM* in one long exhalation. After this exhalation the sound disappears in silence.

Follow the sound with an attentive mind all the way into silence.

Repeat this exercise three times, starting again at the crown of your head. Try to simultaneously remain grounded in the bottom of the bowl.

Repeat this exercise another three times.

❀ Next, start your inhale from a point one-and-a-half feet above your head. Imagine this as a source of brilliant white light.

Visualize your outbreath as a river of white light flowing down your spine into your bowl (see figure 5.6). This bowl transforms into a sea of white light.

Again, silently let the *HUUU* flow into an *MMM* . . . Repeat this breath a number of times. This *MMM* fills your bowl until it really becomes a sea of white light.

Then there is just silence. The only thing left is the smile around your lips. You become that smile.

Quiet all sound and sit silently for a few moments, keeping all your awareness in the flow of your breath and other sensations in your body.

Keep your awareness in the present moment. Stabilize it in the here and now.

Let it expand more and more into the infinite space of the here and now.

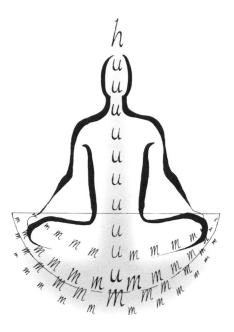

*Figure 5.6. Move your breath in the form of a river
of brilliant white light from above your head, down your spine,
to fill the sea of your pelvic bowl.*

✳ Visualization

Sit straight in a chair or cross-legged or in half-lotus on a cushion on the floor.

Visualize three centers of energy in your body as radiant lights.

The first center is the empty space in the middle of your pelvic bowl, right in front of your sacrum.

The second center is situated at the bottom of your bowl, one-and-a-half feet beneath your pelvic floor.

The third center is one-and-a-half feet above your head.

Visualize simultaneously the bowl and a fine but strong

thread of white light right through your spinal column connecting these three centers.

Sit relaxed and observe your breath.

❀ Inhale through your sacrum and try to sense how you receive cosmic energy.

Exhale down your body and imagine how you receive boundless energy from the center of light one-and-a-half feet above your head. This flow of energy connects with the center of energy one-and-a-half feet beneath you and continues further down into the earth (see figure 5.7).

This way of breathing cleanses and strengthens the energy field within and around your body in a very effective and powerful way.

Meditate in this way for a few more minutes.

Remain in this position. Observe all the sensations in a detached way. Keep your attention open, relaxed, and clear, even when any sensations are intense.

◄■►

Inevitably, every sensation and emotion will change in character. Everything that appears will eventually disappear in the way it exists in this moment. Even intense pain, fear, or anger consist of a series of appearing and disappearing moments, continuously arising and ceasing.

Your bowl helps you to allow and accept everything that arises with compassion.

Your straight spine helps you to face everything, whatever it is, with courage.

Sitting with a straight spine also helps you to "see it through" and to literally see through it.

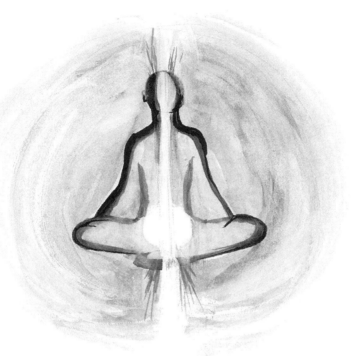

Figure 5.7. Connecting the energy above your head and beneath your sacrum through the breath cleanses and strengthens the energy field within and around your body.

You may also see how everything disappears and dissolves in empty space, and you may see empty space in the heart of everything.

Eventually you may feel the bliss of observing how your sense of being a separate, independent, permanent ego appears and how it disappears when you have the patience and the courage to see through it, seeing empty space in its heart, open and compassionate.

This exercise can have a powerful healing effect on two levels. It can heal physical and emotional pain, even disease. On a deeper level it can heal the sickness of ego: our disconnecting and fragmenting mind.

🧘 Back to Buddha's Basic
Breathing Meditation

Let go of all the images.

Let go of all the promises and expectations that may have been created by the above words.

Return to the simplicity of the basic breathing exercise. Completely empty your mind of thoughts and words.

Let your mind be filled with the breath. Let it be silent.

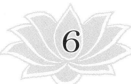

The Open Heart
Being in Love Again

What a remarkable pilgrimage this is! The country you left was your old me. The borders you crossed were those of your ego mind. This pilgrimage took you nowhere and everywhere at the same time. It took you into the wide open space of the here and now. It put you in touch with reality in ways you may have never touched before, imprisoned as you have been in your own dualistic and conceptual mind.

Unlike the ancient Greek king Croesus, whose touch turned everything into lifeless gold, everything you touch turns into living experience. And you touch reality through all of your faculties. This makes you extremely sensitive and sensuous, your senses being wide open. They receive without distortion. Your sight, smell, hearing, taste, and touch are clear, giving true information. Your emotions are sound, strong, and natural, not dictated by your ego's desires, fears, and whims.

Above all, your heart is wide open, in touch with everything and everybody, touching all humans and even all living beings: seeing, hearing, feeling their hearts and minds, their joys and pains, their suffering and their deeply buried potential for bliss. You understand clearly that their deepest suffering is connected with their unconscious fear of bliss, as experiencing bliss means being empty of ego. Bliss results from having had the courage to let go of the ego.

And you suffer for them, although your way of suffering is different from theirs. Their suffering comes from not being in touch with life's impermanence, from fearing and stubbornly resisting this impermanence, always clinging to some dream. They suffer because their minds and hearts are closed. You "went out of your mind," so to speak, and you now suffer because your heart is so wide open, so touched by the suffering you see around you. You suffer because you have the bliss of a heart so open that it can be moved by everything. There is so much space in your heart that you can accommodate the suffering you see around you. You can allow it in; you do not have to push it out. You do not have to protect yourself against it. The bliss of a truly open heart is that it does not need to defend itself against the pain and suffering of another human being.

Once you no longer need distance between you and others, you will have become compassionate.

This kind of compassion is not a virtue of the mind. It is an inescapable consequence of being in touch with reality as it is. Compassion requires first of all liberation from the deadly confines of the ego. It arises out of the joy of your being and penetrating insight into reality, evaporating the cloud of ignorance that sets you apart from the world around you. Ego is nothing more than the distance it continuously creates and stubbornly defends. Therefore, ego can never be truly compassionate. It may seem compassionate, but then it is lying.

Compassion requires the greatest courage: the courage to leave the ego's safe, defensive fortress. It requires going out into this world to meet life and death and becoming truly intimate with the joys and suffering of humankind.

You need all of this courage and compassion in order to practice the highest meditation. In the Tibetan school of Mahayana Buddhism this is called *Tonglen:* giving and taking. The Dalai Lama explains this meditation as "visualizing taking upon yourself all the suffering, pain, negativity, and undesirable experiences of other sentient beings. You imagine taking these upon yourself and then giving away or sharing with others your own positive qualities."

The journey has come full circle. The nitty-gritty of daily life that you had wanted to leave—this world full of misery, pain, and injustice—is here again. Right in front of you and all around you. All the things and people you wanted to escape you now embrace.

So now, when you breathe out you really let yourself go into the pain and suffering of the people around you. And when you breathe in you let their pain and suffering come into your heart. Breathing this way helps the final breaking of the heart, the final breakthrough of the light through the defensive walls of your ego mind. This is the ultimate spiritual adventure and the ultimate spiritual discovery: that in the breaking of the heart, the deepest bliss and the highest ecstasy lie. For a broken heart is an open heart, and only an open heart has the space that includes everything: all of life and every living being. The ecstasy of a broken heart is born from being in the heart of humankind, in the middle of life. This is truly being in love.

It is the same ecstasy that Jesus experienced on the top of Mount Tabor, radiating light in all directions, touching everything and everybody, encompassing all of life, embracing all humankind's suffering.

In that one moment on Mount Tabor all of his life came to a climax. The past and the future merged. The distances between the moments of his birth, his death, and his resurrection vanished.

To the bewilderment of his three closest disciples, his whole body turned into a blazing light, the power of pure immaculate consciousness, a consciousness that compassionately encompassed the whole world and the entire universe.

With the exercise in this chapter we have reached our Mount Tabor. Here we experience the climax of all the previous exercises. Now your own body can transform into a space filled with light radiating in all directions.

The Open Heart

🧘 Buddha's Basic Breathing Meditation

Find a comfortable position and follow ten cycles of breathing with full attentiveness.

🧘 Meditative Breathing Exercises

When you breathe in, observe how clean, fresh air enters through your nose while at the same time cosmic energy enters your body through your sacrum.

Let the breath naturally move through the whole sacred space of your body when you breathe in and out.

Leave space for silence.

✳ Breath-Body Movement

OPENING THE HEART OF COURAGE AND COMPASSION

Sit straight on a chair or cross-legged or in half-lotus on a cushion on the floor.

Connect with the earth beneath you through the triangle of your two sitting bones and your tailbone.

Root the triangle with a warm orange color (see figure 6.1 on page 70).

Generate the bowl, visualize it, and let it become a living experience.

Generate the energy center in the middle of the bowl.

Generate the thread of white light in the middle of your spinal column.

Generate the energy field within and around your body (see figure 6.2 on page 70).

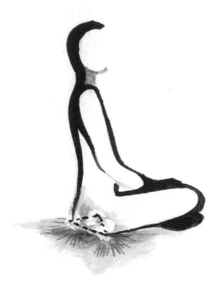

Figure 6.1. Connect with the earth beneath through the
triangle formed by your two sitting bones and your tailbone.

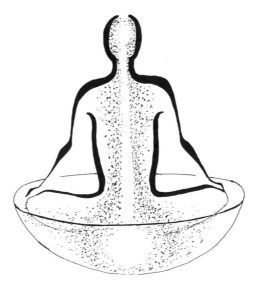

Figure 6.2. Generate the energy of the pelvic bowl
within your body.

✻ Inhale and raise your arms, spreading them sideways to the right and left. Continue moving them upward until you touch your hands together as if in a center of radiant white light culminating approximately one-and-a-half feet above your head.

While you do this, imagine that you gather boundless energy from the space around you.

Exhale and bring your hands down with palms together in a vertical line in front of your body. Energy as brilliant white light descends from the center of white light above your head, flowing down your spine, and into the wide-open bowl.

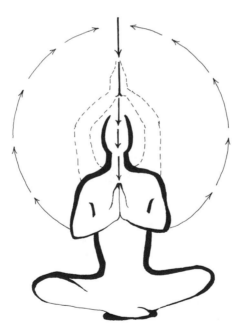

Figure 6.3. Inhale your arms out to the sides,
letting palms meet overhead as if in a circle of radiant white light.
Exhale with hands together down the front of your body,
drawing brilliant white light down through your spine.

You may attribute to this white light any quality that you need most at the present moment. Healing . . . patience . . . joy . . .

Or you might just wait and see what happens spontaneously and what energy quality comes to you.

Repeat three times . . .

🌼 Rest your hands on your thighs with palms turned up and fingers pointing toward the center of your pelvic bowl.

Breathe in, let your hands come together in front of your body, and raise them with palms together up until they reach the center of energy and light above your head.

Breathe out and lower your arms sideways until your hands come to rest again on your thighs.

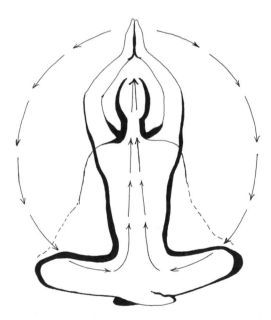

Figure 6.4. Breathe in as your hands rise through your midline and breathe out as they lower to your sides.

Let one breathing cycle pass by and stay relaxed.

Repeat three times . . .

❋ Breathe in and raise your hands from the center of your bowl toward your heart in prayer position.

Breathe out and spread your arms to the right and left, opening your heart toward the world around you.

The arms come down again in the breathing pause.

Stay relaxed and let one breathing cycle pass.

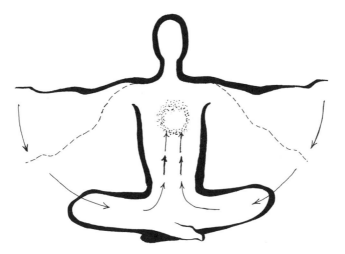

Figure 6.5. Bring your hands to your heart and then open them toward the world around you.

Repeat three times . . .

❋ Sound

Rise and stand with your feet a little apart from each other. Root them firmly into the earth beneath you. Connect with your center of earth energy one-and-a-half feet beneath your feet.

Breathe in and raise your hands upward until they reach the center of energy as white light one-and-a-half feet above your head.

Imagine that you hear the sound *OM* come to you, bringing with it boundless, positive, and healing energy from the space around you.

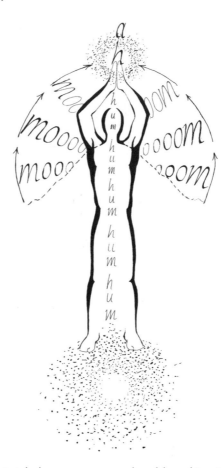

Figure 6.6. Inhale your arms overhead breathing in OM. Hold your breath with AH. Exhale your hands down the center of your body, palms together, with the sound HUM.

Hold your breath for a moment with a silent *AH*.

Breathe out and bring your hands down with palms together in a vertical line in front of your body. Let the sound *HUM* softly reverberate in you while you do this.

Stay relaxed and let one breathing cycle pass.

Repeat three times . . .

✳ Visualization

ON A HIGH MOUNTAIN—MOUNT TABOR

You can do this exercise seated or standing up.

Visualize yourself standing on a high mountain such as Mount Tabor in Galilee, where Jesus was transfigured and manifested the essence of his human-divine being in a radiant light.

Your feet are firmly rooted in the earth. You have a clear view all around. The sky above is blue and cloudless. The sun is warm.

Breathe in and experience receiving light and boundless healing energy while at the same time, out of the universe, the silent sound *OM* comes to you and fills you completely.

Hold your breath and experience bringing it all in with a silent *AH*. Enjoy the feeling of this moment.

Breathe out and experience giving it all in a silent *HUM*.

Stay relaxed and experience . . . silence.

Let one breathing cycle pass and experience the silence filling with the sound of *OM* when you breathe in.

Hold your breath and enjoy the energy in silent bliss—*AH*.

Breathe out and radiate this blissful energy as a healing light in all directions—*HUM.*

OM, AH, HUM should come back again. It is the basic form of all mantras.

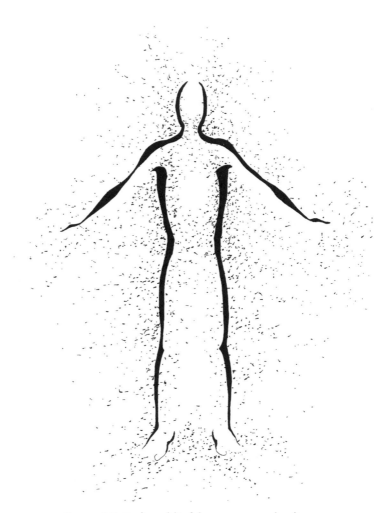

Figure 6.7. Radiate blissful energy as a healing and consoling light in all directions.

IN THE VALLEY OF THIS WORLD—GOLGOTHA

In this exercise we go against our instincts and experiment with doing the opposite of what we are inclined to do, which is to avoid suffering and seek pleasure. This practice incorporates Tonglen (receiving and giving), a meditation practice found in Mahayana Buddhism.

◄■►

Again, you can do this exercise either seated or standing.

Visualize yourself standing in the middle of the world, as if it is a Golgotha, where Jesus was crucified and met his physical death. Realize the pain and suffering of this world and open your heart to it.

It may be the suffering of one single person you love or the suffering of many millions in distant places. It may also be your own suffering on this particular day.

Breathe in with a silent *OM* and visualize receiving the suffering of others entering your heart in the form of black smoke.

Hold your breath with a silent *AH* and visualize the suffering of others entering your heart, effectively destroying all the clinging and self-cherishing of your own ego mind. Let the suffering you see break your heart, and because of this you break through to the great compassion and love found in the depths of your heart.

Breathe out with a silent *HUM* and radiate this compassion and love as white healing light and energy to those who need this.

Be silent now and visualize how this light fills and heals yourself and others in body, mind, and soul.

Enjoy having the courage and compassion to do this exercise.

🧘 Adaptation of Buddha's Basic Breathing Meditation

I AM THE ALPHA AND THE OMEGA—AOM

As in Buddha's Basic Breathing Meditation, sit quietly and observe your breath.

Breathe in silently.

Hold the breath a moment.

Breathe out and—silently—let the sound *AHHHH* and *OOO* melt into *HUMMM . . .*

AHH . . . OOO . . . HUU . . . MMM . . .

Experience how all the opposites and contradictions of life melt into One.

At the same time you are both on top of a high mountain and in the valley of this world. In this same moment you are fully living and dying, suffering and rejoicing.

In this very moment you are experiencing everything implied by the names Tabor (glorious transfiguration) and Golgotha (suffering and death).

Buddha's Basic Breathing Meditation is unexpectedly Christian!

PART 3

· · · · · · ·

BREATH, BODY, AND ACTION

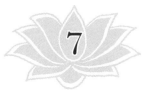

7

Acting

Healing the World by Touch

As much as you wanted to escape this world before is as much as you now want to stay.

The truth is that you cannot escape this world, however much you'd like to. You realize that you are an inescapable part of it. The oppressive and confining feeling this once caused you has disappeared, however. It disappeared because you broke your heart, and this broken heart opened you to everything and everybody in a very radical way. You now "wholeheartedly" turn to this world and relate to it with the open heart of a bodhisattva.

A bodhisattva has a heart that is radically turned to this world. Such a person vows to not enter the final blissful state of nirvana as long as the last blade of grass is not free. He or she may seem not "of this world," but such a person is definitely *in* this world. The bodhisattva's open heart that turns to this world and not away from it is very much like Jesus's coming down Mount Tabor to continue his journey to Jerusalem. He did not allow his disciples to stay much longer on the top of Mount Tabor as if they wanted to hold on to that special moment. He did not remain on the mountain in his transfigured state, but instead he went back to the world, where the first thing he did was to heal a sick man who was possessed by a powerful evil spirit. And the last thing he did was to heal humankind.

According to the gospels as well as the teachings of the Buddha, this is the way every man and woman must go. It is everyone's final destiny to be healed and to heal others. In the Mahayana tradition of Buddhism this is called the bodhisattva's way of life. A bodhisattva is not necessarily Buddhist, such a person can profess any religious affiliation—Judiasm, Christianity, Islam—or be an atheist. A bodhisattva can be a man or a woman, young or old.

Renouncing the blissful state of individual enlightenment is not the sacrifice some might take it for. It is the true and logical consequence of having an open heart.

A bodhisattva experiences no joy in partial rejoicing. She or he sees no light in individual enlightenment. The bliss that comes with personal enlightenment is not enough for bodhisattvas because individual enlightenment does not include everything and everybody. For the bodhisattva true enlightenment wants to penetrate every dark corner of this universe, and real bliss must touch everything that exists.

It is in the nature of a bodhisattva to naturally want to touch, heal, and liberate everything and everybody. The bodhisattva wants to change this world not out of political ambition or a religious mission, but because it is the bodhisattva's nature to want to dispel darkness and alleviate suffering. The bodhisattva does this first by being whole-heartedly devoted to this world and truly part of it.

A bodhisattva acts but is not agitated.

She works but is not driven.

He speaks his mind but is not rude or insulting.

She convinces by her manner.

He is quiet but not timid.

She is relaxed, yet many things get done.

He sees clearly how much suffering is caused by human injustice and ignorance, but never turns violent against the oppressors.

A bodhisattva is creative, intelligent, flexible, effective, and patient.

She expresses herself in myriad forms, lifestyles, and professions: as a doctor, an artist, a teacher, a mother, and more.

A bodhisattva betrays himself by his touch because his kind of enlightenment is not only of his mind, but also of his body, and especially of his hands. One recognizes a bodhi-sattva by the way he shakes your hand, caresses a baby, comforts a patient, and even by the way he makes love.

The touch of her hands is soft yet firm. Her hands feel warm and supportive. They always convey a sense of holding, never one of pushing, pulling, or grasping. A bodhisattva puts her whole heart in her touch and therefore knows how to touch the heart of another person. She also puts a pure mind in her touch, and therefore her touch is always safe and trustworthy. Her touch is never manipulative, seductive, or directive.

A bodhisattva loves to work with his hands, massaging,

cooking, painting, playing an instrument, gardening, etc. A bodhisattva can't help but be a healer, because he channels energies that come from the depths of his being and from the universe itself.

If you want to find out if you've met a bodhisattva, shake hands with him or her. Shake hands with a politician, and that handshake will tell you whether this person is motivated by greed for power or by compassion. You know immediately whether you'd want to vote for him or her. In the same way you know by what doctor you want to be treated and by what lover caressed.

If you want to become a bodhisattva, put your whole heart and a pure mind into your hands. Reach out to touch and heal this world. Don't withdraw your hands and your heart from the pain and suffering of this world. It makes no sense, as suffering is the First Noble Truth about life in this world.

Healing the World by Touch

🧘 *Buddha's Basic Breathing Meditation*

Find a comfortable position and follow ten cycles of breathing with full attentiveness.

🧘 *Meditative Breathing Exercises*

Observe the movement of your breath within and around the center of your pelvic bowl. Realize that the breath enters your body through your nose and at the same time, as a current of energy, through the sacrum and the pores of your skin all over your body.

✳ Breath-Body Movement

Sit straight in a chair or cross-legged or in half-lotus on a cushion on the floor.

Feel yourself well connected with the earth beneath you.

Generate the bowl (see figure 7.1).

Generate the white light in its center.

Generate the thread of white light through your spine.

Generate the energy field within and around your body.

Open your heart of courage and compassion.

Put your left hand in your lap with the palm turned upward.

Put your right hand on your right knee with the palm turned upward and the fingers close together (see figure 7.2 on page 86).

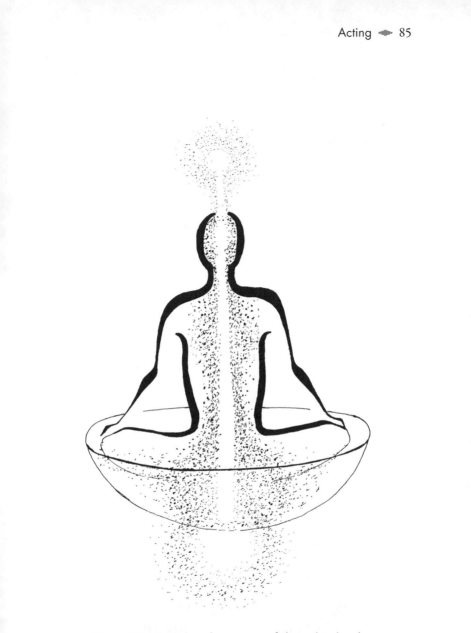

Figure 7.1. Generate the energy of the pelvic bowl within your body.

Open the center of your right hand by slightly extending the fingers. Imagine a beam of rich golden light radiating from this hand. Discover how this image affects your whole being. Be aware of all the sensations and feelings that arise. Give them space.

You may increase the feeling by slightly extending the joints of your right wrist and your fingers.

Slightly extend the joint of your right elbow.

Slightly extend the joint of your right shoulder.

Slightly extend your spinal column.

Widen the bowl and strengthen its center of white light.

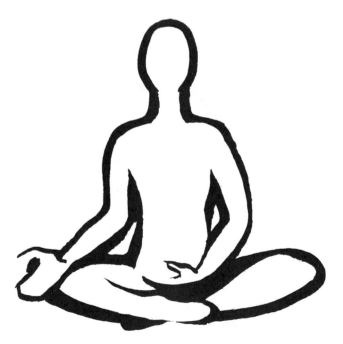

Figure 7.2. With palms turned upward, left hand in your lap and right hand on your right knee, allow a beam of rich golden light to radiate from your right palm.

How does the feeling change you and the sense you have of yourself?

Relax your body now and sit in a way that feels comfortable to you.

Your left hand, still lying in your lap, is on the side of the heart and reinforces the energy of giving from the heart, an energy that will eventually flow through both hands.

Try to keep the flow of feeling that this exercise created in you while you visualize yourself engaged in some of your daily activities, such as cooking, gardening, massaging somebody, holding a baby, or hugging a loved one.

Meditation in Action

Experiment with the flow of feelings created in the previous exercise during your daily activities, especially when you touch people, whether comforting, making love, or just shaking hands. As well, experiment with these feelings when you touch objects you care for, such as flowers, food, etc. You can even experiment with it when you touch money, practicing giving instead of grasping.

Heal the world with your touch.

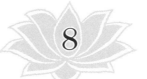

Speaking

Healing the World by Speech

A bodhisattva is recognized by the way she speaks. Her words are true because she speaks from the truth, being deeply in touch with true life.

In a bodhisattva's words the truth comes alive. He brings it out in every situation. Truth starts to move, breathe, and reverberate wherever a bodhisattva appears.

The truth reacts immediately when it hears the voice of the bodhisattva. It rises to the surface and breaks through the layers that covered it.

The voice of a bodhisattva has something magical. It has the same magic as the kiss of the prince who awakened the Sleeping Beauty from her hundred years' slumber. The voice of a bodhisattva has the magic power to kiss the truth back to life. At the same time it has the penetrating power to cut through the layers of lies that hide the truth. A bodhisattva cannot help but expose all phoniness and falseness. Just as the bodhisattva once had the courage to step out of the world of lies, she now has the courage to step into the truth of a situation. And the painful truth is that this world is full of lies, and people's minds are filled with the many lies that they tell themselves and one another. Living in their mental clouds of hopes, fears, and fantasies, not in touch with the truth of their own lives, most people do not know how many lies they tell. A bodhisattva is therefore an uneasy comrade. He is a prince, a lover, and a revolutionary. You feel attracted to him and repulsed by him. You want to listen to him and silence him. You want the kiss from his lips and to shut his mouth forever.

We all spoke with the voice of a bodhisattva when we were children, saying out loud everything we felt and thought.

We stopped speaking like bodhisattvas as soon as we realized that we had to say the things that were expected of us. Soon we became accomplices in the adult world of lies. We gave up on speaking the truth out of the sheer need to survive emotionally, to belong and to not be left alone. It was not out of cowardice, but out of a need for love that we stopped speaking the truth. And after we had been silent long enough we finally lost touch with the truth. We forgot . . .

We became part of the all-pervasive ignorance.

The voice of a bodhisattva is able to pierce through this cloud of ignorance and touch the heart of the child we once were.

The power behind the speech of a bodhisattva is born from a deep inner silence that sounds right through his words and his voice.

A bodhisattva has no need to say much. Therefore she is

free to really listen. It can be said that one can recognize a bodhisattva by her way of listening. It's very much like her quality of touching. Her listening is a way of deeply touching you, accepting you completely as you are, yet supporting your potential to become more yourself.

One can master the speech of a bodhisattva by making listening a daily practice. Cultivating the art of listening is very much like cultivating the art of meditation. As in meditation, it is silently attending to what presents itself without interrupting, commenting on, or arguing with what one hears.

Similarly, as silence is the mother of all sound, silently listening is the mother of all speech.

Practicing listening like a bodhisattva can have many practical implications in daily life—in the office, the hospital, or in your own home.

It is essential that you do your own listening experiments and discover the effects for yourself. Notice the difference in the way the other person honestly reveals more of himself or herself. Also notice differences in what you yourself say and how you say it. Experience the difference in responding from real, silent listening, in contrast to responding from a precoded set of questions and answers. This kind of silent listening and responding involves "letting yourself go," and like going on a journey into a foreign country, it requires quite a bit of courage. It also requires a lot of compassion, as you know how much pain and fear can come free when the truth is touched and the lies are laid bare.

So listening is a pilgrimage out of the known and familiar into the unknown space of a true encounter with another person.

A bodhisattva is compassionate, as she has the sensitivity of a child. Like a child she is easily touched and hurt. But where a child has to stop feeling so much pain, a bodhisattva goes on, having the strength to suffer the pain. She does not withdraw into the silence of adulthood. Her most powerful weapon may be that she is very honest about her pain and having her heart broken. She has the courage to speak out, to sometimes cry out, and to show publicly what often is suffered in secret. This is no show of cheap and socially acceptable indignation, but a showing of the wounds that one incurs when the truth is betrayed.

This is a holy drama, and a bodhisattva is a holy actor. He is a child, a saint, and a warrior. She is a crazy mother in Argentina, a crying nun in Lhasa, a student in front of a tank in Beijing.

Healing the World with Speech

· ·

🧘 Buddha's Basic Breathing Meditation

Find a comfortable position and follow ten cycles of breathing with full attentiveness.

🧘 Meditative Breathing Exercises

Sit straight on a chair or cross-legged or in half-lotus on a cushion on the floor. Feel yourself well connected with the earth beneath you.

Generate the bowl (see figure 8.1).

Generate a center within the space of the bowl, visualizing it as white light.

Generate a thread of this white light through your spinal column and connect this with a center of white light one-and-a-half feet above your head and underneath your pelvis.

Generate the energy field within and around your body.

Open your heart of courage and compassion.

Put your right hand on your right knee with palm turned upward.

After a little while put your left hand on your left knee, also with the palm turned upward. Let both hands rest relaxed, open, and receptive (see figure 8.2).

Feel the connection between your hands and the bowl of your pelvis . . . your heart . . . the back of your head.

Let this posture open your ears and the space between your ears inside your head. Let this open your hearing.

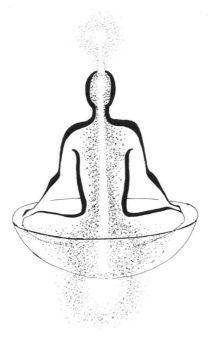

Figure 8.1. Generate the energy of the pelvic bowl
within and around your body.

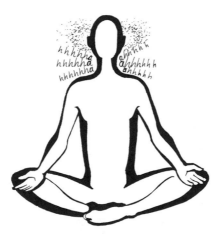

Figure 8.2. Sit straight on a chair or cross-legged or
in half-lotus, with your hands open on your knees.

Experiment with pure hearing, without judging or interpreting. Listen to sounds, street noises, voices.

Sit quietly breathing in and out.

Now place the back of your right hand in the palm of your left hand.

Experiment with listening to the sounds within yourself. Listen to the silence within.

Listen for an inner voice. If you don't hear an inner voice, content yourself with listening to the silence.

Sit quietly, breathing in and out.

Breathe out an *AHHH* . . . Let your vocal cords vibrate with the sound. Let the sound become soft, strong, and clear. Let it resonate in the space of your body.

Let your voice be healed. Let your voice be healing.

Experiment with speaking with this voice while you read or recite a poem, sing a song, or say a prayer.

🧘 Meditation in Action

Experiment with the physical and mental space of listening throughout the day. Let your speech come from this spacious quality of listening. Respond to what you really hear, outside and within you . . .

With compassion.

With courage.

Heal the world through your speech.

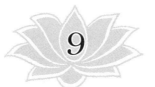

Being Silent

Healing the World by Being Present

The main characteristic of a bodhisattva is her quality of presence, meaning she is fully present in the here and now. This presence is tender, modest, and powerful at the same time. It has a quality of nakedness, as it is not dressed in impressive or outstanding characteristics. A bodhisattva has no personality that draws the attention of TV cameras. A bodhisattva has no personality in the sense of a set of closely knitted character traits that hide one's inner being. She may therefore be difficult to discover and even more difficult to relate to, as she does not give you an easy handle to get ahold of her.

You cannot push or pull a bodhisattva. If you want to hit him, it's as if you're striking thin air. If you want to insult him, there seems to be nobody there to be insulted. And if you want to love him, he eludes all the possessive clinging that love so often entails.

Yet a bodhisattva is very much present. She is there when you just decided to give up on her and you stopped loving, fearing, or looking for her. If she is there, you feel yourself

surrounded by a loving presence, a kind of energy that you
can only feel after you become quiet of wanting it. It's a healing energy in the truest sense, as it heals the divisive actions
of the mind. It's an energy that fills the fissures and gaps in
the heart of humankind. A bodhisattva brings peace into this
world not as a political solution, but as a living experience.
She is a grassroots peacekeeper, kind yet fearless.

A bodhisattva brings light into this world not out of a
crusade against the dark and evil forces, but out of the sheer
joy of radiating his true essence in all directions and in every
situation.

A bodhisattva brings healing into this world not out of
fear of sickness and death, but out of bringing people back to
their true nature, their original pureness: the inner light of
their own soul, heart, and mind.

The yoga of courage and compassion is in fact a pilgrimage to arrive at this inner light and to become a "light unto
this world." It is not a pilgrimage to visit some holy place or
meet a holy man. It's all about becoming your own true self:
becoming a bodhisattva. It's about becoming Buddha, becoming Christ. It's simply about becoming a real person.

As long as we do not have the courage to cross the distance that separates us from a bodhisattva, from Buddha and
Christ, we remain imprisoned in our own dualistic mind. As
long as we do not have the courage and the power to break
through the walls that separate the Buddha and the Christ,
Buddhism and Christianity, East and West, north and south,
peace will not have a chance. As long as we need to pre-
serve our cherished identities of being so different from one
another—Jew, Muslim, Hindu, Christian, Buddhist—we

shall never be able to identify our deepest, innermost nature. In the depths of our being we are all brothers and sisters, we are all One. Only from the depths of our being can we be truly loving and compassionate.

To become One is the final goal of our pilgrimage. Only then will peace have a chance. Inner peace and world peace will then be fundamentally one and the same, as the one (inner peace) cannot possibly exist without the other (world peace). In the depths of our being we are one another's brothers and sisters. We are all One.

This may still seem a distant ideal, but it's the only option for our survival as a human race.

True peacekeeping means training our bodies and minds in such a way that peace becomes a living experience, the most precious gift from our souls.

This yoga of courage and compassion may guide your way into and right through your body mind in order to experience the inner light of peace. It may then help you to guide this inner light out into the world, until the last blade of grass is touched by you.

Healing the World by Being Present

🧘 Buddha's Basic Breathing Meditation

Find a comfortable position and follow ten cycles of breathing with full attentiveness.

🧘 Meditative Breathing Exercises

Sit straight on a chair or cross-legged or in half-lotus on a cushion on the floor.

Feel yourself well connected with the earth beneath you.

Place your right hand in your left palm. The tips of your thumbs lightly touch each other.

The tip of your tongue lightly touches your palate just behind the front teeth.

Generate the bowl.

Generate the center within the space of the bowl. Visualize it radiating white light.

Generate a thread of white light through your spinal column, connected to the energy centers above the head and at the bottom of the bowl.

Generate the energy field within and around your body.

Open your heart of courage and compassion.

Visualize a beautiful, soft white light in the spot between and a little above your eyes.

Feel an inner connection between the light in the center of your bowl and the light between your eyes.

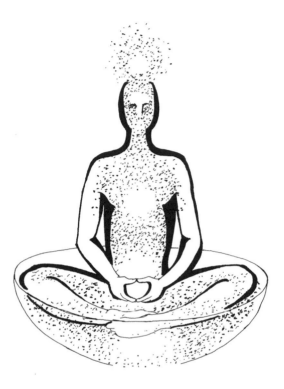

Figure 9.1. Feel an inner connection between the light in the center of your bowl and the light between your eyes.

Breathe in and go with your attention from within the center of your bowl, through your spine, over the midline of your head, and into the space between your eyes.

Stop there for a brief moment.

Breathe out and go with your attention downward—down your nose, tongue, throat, chest, stomach, belly, bowl, and into its center.

Silently make the sounds *OM . . . AH . . . HUM . . .*

OM breathing in, *AH* pausing in the space between your eyes, *HUM* breathing out.

Repeat seven times . . .

Relax and, with a soft inner smile, let the light between your eyes quietly spread over your face . . . into your head . . . down your shoulders, down your arms, filling your chest, filling your belly and bowl . . . spreading into your legs, feet, and toes. Spreading beyond your body, filling the room you are in . . . your house . . . the street . . .

Let it spread as far as it naturally goes, entering all the dark corners, anywhere there is suffering . . . alleviating, transforming, enlightening.

🧘 Meditation in Action

Experiment with this living, transforming light wherever you are, whatever you do, whomever you are with.

Heal the world by your presence.

Index